Nabila Kalla
Ouanassa Hamouda

COVID-19 infection in healthcare workers

Nabila Kalla
Ouanassa Hamouda

COVID-19 infection in healthcare workers

ScienciaScripts

Imprint
Any brand names and product names mentioned in this book are subject to trademark, brand or patent protection and are trademarks or registered trademarks of their respective holders. The use of brand names, product names, common names, trade names, product descriptions etc. even without a particular marking in this work is in no way to be construed to mean that such names may be regarded as unrestricted in respect of trademark and brand protection legislation and could thus be used by anyone.

Cover image: www.ingimage.com

This book is a translation from the original published under ISBN 978-3-639-62408-3.

Publisher:
Sciencia Scripts
is a trademark of
Dodo Books Indian Ocean Ltd. and OmniScriptum S.R.L publishing group

120 High Road, East Finchley, London, N2 9ED, United Kingdom
Str. Armeneasca 28/1, office 1, Chisinau MD-2012, Republic of Moldova, Europe
Managing Directors: Ieva Konstantinova, Victoria Ursu
info@omniscriptum.com

Printed at: see last page
ISBN: 978-620-8-39950-4

Copyright © Nabila Kalla, Ouanassa Hamouda
Copyright © 2024 Dodo Books Indian Ocean Ltd. and OmniScriptum S.R.L publishing group

COVID-19 infection in healthcare workers

Table of contents :

1. Introduction:

In December 2019, an outbreak of dyspnea pneumonia of undetermined cause was discovered in Wuhan, China. This enabled Chinese researchers to quickly identify the cause of the disease in January 2020. In February 2020, the World Health Organisation (WHO) named the disease linked to this virus covid-19. Initially, the virus was called nCoV-2019, then renamed SARS-CoV-2 by a group of experts in virus classification.

Covid-19 infection is a viral pathology. It can present as a simple flu-like syndrome, pneumonia in some cases, or acute respiratory distress syndrome, which is the most serious form of the disease.

Covid-19 began at the end of 2019 in China. This infection had a big impact on the world and health, leading to millions of deaths. It was a global health crisis, prompting officials to prioritise the search for a real solution to curb its emergence.

In Algeria, the first case was reported on 25 February 2020. It involved an Italian living in a camp at Hassi Messaoud, in the town of Ouargla. In March, several people were infected with the virus in the town of Blida.

Efforts have been made by researchers to develop treatments and vaccines aimed primarily at combating covid-19. Vaccination of the Algerian population began in January 2021. Carers were given priority for vaccination.

During this covid-19 pandemic, healthcare workers represent the population most exposed to the risk of contamination by SARS-COV 2

. Healthcare professionals are still on the front line in the fight against the covid-19 pandemic. Covid-19 infection in healthcare workers poses a real problem in healthcare facilities, with absenteeism among infected staff having an impact on better patient care. It is therefore essential to identify the various potential risk factors for contamination, in order to combat nosocomial covid and try to develop appropriate prevention strategies.

The aim of this study was to determine the prevalence and main risk factors for covid-19 infection among healthcare workers working in hospital units dedicated to the care of patients infected with SARS - CoV 2.

The aim of this work is also to describe :

- The particularities of covid-19 infection in healthcare professionals caring for patients with covid-19.
- Acceptance of the SARS COV-2 vaccine among healthcare professionals.
- The vaccination coverage rate for healthcare professionals working in covid-19 patient care units.

2. Virology :

SARS-CoV-2 is a single-stranded RNA virus. SARS-CoV-2 is a coarsely spherical enveloped virus ranging in size from 80 to 200 nm in diameter. The envelope of this virus is composed of the surface protein S, which is arranged in a corona, hence the name "corona". It is one of the largest genomes of RNA viruses infecting humans.

3. Contamination :

SARS-CoV-2 is spread mainly by respiratory droplets. These droplets containing particles of the virus can infect a vulnerable person either by direct contamination of a mucous membrane, or by touching a surface contaminated by nasal, oral or ocular secretions (indirect contamination). They can be expelled several metres, but do not remain in the atmosphere for long. On the other hand, the virus can remain alive for several days on non-living surfaces.

You risk developing the disease by handling surfaces infected with the virus before touching areas of the face such as the eyes, nose or mouth. Under the right conditions, the virus can remain in the air for up to three hours, on cardboard for up to 24 hours, and for up to two or three days on plastic and stainless steel.

With regard to maternal-foetal transmission, higher levels of antibodies and abnormal levels of cytokines were observed in a newborn baby whose mother had had covid-19. Tests carried out 2 hours after birth showed that the baby had received the virus during pregnancy, but not through the placenta.

A recent study found traces of the virus in the breast milk of breast-feeding mothers. Given that the sample was limited, it would be beneficial to carry out studies on a larger sample size in order to identify this mode of transmission more quickly.

4. Clinical :

4.1 . Clinical signs :

SARS-CoV enters the body's cells via the angiotensin-converting enzyme. After an incubation period of around five days, symptoms set in, varying in severity and expression from one individual to another, ranging from mild to severe.

The risk of developing serious complications or dying as a result of covid-19 increases with age, tobacco consumption, and in individuals suffering from severe medical conditions such as cancer, heart, lung, kidney or liver disease, diabetes, reduced immunity, sickle cell disease or obesity.

Most cases of Covid-19 result in lung disease, accompanied by a variety of symptoms:

- Fever
- Rhinorrhea
- Pharyngitis
- Dyspnoea
- Cough
- Chest pain

Certain symptoms frequently associated with fevers, such as headaches, muscle aches, chills and sweating, were also noted.

Some individuals infected with covid-19 report digestive problems such as nausea, vomiting, diarrhoea and stomach pains. In some individuals, symptoms of diarrhoea and nausea appear before the onset of fever and respiratory signs.

The frequent presence of problems with the sense of smell (anosmia) or a reduction in the sense of smell (hyposmia), as well as the loss of taste (agueusia) or a reduction in taste (hypogueusia) has attracted the attention of doctors. They are wondering how these signs can be useful in making common diagnoses.

In the case of covid-19, the dermatological problems are inflammatory, such as erythema, vesicles and urticaria, but also vascular, resulting in purplish patches, livedo, purpura, chilblains and angiomas. They could be due to an excessive inflammatory response.

Difficulty breathing can occur between the fifth and eighth day. This often leads to people being admitted to hospital (on average after 7 days), but sometimes it is not accompanied by a drop in oxygen or rapid breathing.

The severity of the disease is manifested by breathing difficulties, low oxygenation and considerable injury detected during lung imaging examinations. This can lead to breathing difficulties requiring mechanical assistance to breathe, shock, complications in various organs and can even lead to death.

The main complication is acute respiratory distress syndrome, which occurs in 20% of patients with breathing difficulties, on average 8 days after the onset of their symptoms. This syndrome depends on various factors, making it diverse and difficult to anticipate.

The prognosis is strongly influenced by age, the presence of other illnesses and the general state of health at the time of infection. Acute respiratory distress syndrome (ARDS) in patients can lead to rapid deterioration and a risk of mortality due to multi-organ failure.

Early aggravations are attributed to an increase in viral replication, while later complications are thought to be caused by inflammatory reactions, such as an excessive immune response, which coincide with the production of antibodies.

It has been found that in severe covid-19, the cytokine profile resembles that of secondary haemophagocytic lymphohistiocytosis syndrome, manifested by an increase in certain substances in the body, such as IL-2, IL-7, a factor that helps the formation of granulocytes, and other proteins linked to the immune response and inflammation.

In addition, elevated levels of ferritin and IL-6 may signal an increased risk of mortality, presumably due to excessive inflammation induced by the virus. Based on this, tocilizumab, which inhibits IL-6 receptors, is administered to patients with covid-19 pneumonia and high blood IL-6 levels in order to reduce lung inflammation.

Although coronavirus infection mainly targets the lungs, the presence of ACE2 receptors in various organs can cause problems in the heart, digestive system, kidneys, liver, nerves and eyes, requiring special attention.

The heart and blood vessels are often affected, which can lead to problems such as heart injury, inflammation of the heart muscle, heart attack, heart failure, heart rhythm disorders and blood clots in the veins. A highly sensitive cardiac troponin test is a key element in guiding diagnoses.

Thromboembolic disease is a fairly common complication, which explains the need for specific advice to prevent it with anticoagulant drugs. Clots in deep veins, including those on catheters, and especially plugs in the lungs have been reported. In intensive care, there were more pulmonary embolisms in patients with ARDS due to Covid-19 than in those with ARDS of other causes.

Higher D-dimer levels have been linked to the severity of covid-19. People with severe covid-19 have much higher D-dimer levels than those without the disease. High D-dimer levels may indicate a risk of clotting problems in these patients, who may need treatment to prevent clots from forming.

Nervous problems such as myelitis infections, Guillain-Barré syndrome, acute cerebral infections and brain disorders have been reported.

An inflammatory condition affecting various body systems has been noted as a rare complication of SARS-CoV-2 infection, with features similar to Kawasaki disease or toxic shock syndrome. Children with

MIS-C often have fever, a rapid heart rate, signs of inflammation throughout the body and problems in several organs.
The syndrome can affect the heart, stomach and kidneys 2 to 6 months after an infection, which is generally mild or without symptoms, caused by SARS-CoV-2.
In the majority of patients, symptoms generally disappear within a week. However, some individuals may experience a deterioration in their condition after a week, which could lead to serious illnesses such as acute respiratory distress syndrome. Even patients with moderate illness can have lingering symptoms, such as difficulty breathing, coughing and feeling unwell. These symptoms can last for weeks or even months. Long-lasting illness seems to be more common when the disease is severe.
PCR tests, designed to detect the virus in patients, may continue to give positive results for at least 3 months, even if they show no signs of illness. However, even patients with long-lasting symptoms are not usually seen as contagious, as the virus is almost never found in patients' airways after 10 days of illness.
Covid-19 can also cause health problems that last a long time, even after the illness. Symptoms can remain for months. This has been called by various names, such as long covid or post-covid-19 syndrome, and is thought to affect between 25% and 50% of patients in some studies in the United States.
Cognitive problems, weakness, fatigue, myalgias, pain and dyspnoea are frequently reported. Risks of long-term problems may include a more severe form of the disease, being older, being female and already having lung problems.

Factors increasing the risk of lasting complications include advanced age, female gender, a history of lung problems and a more severe form of the disease.

According to the WHO, covid-19 is classified into three levels of severity.

4.2. Clinical forms:

4.2.1 A severe form of COVID-19 :

is when a person has criteria such as severe difficulty in breathing, severe infection, shock caused by infection, or other health problems that generally require intensive care, such as needing a machine to help them breathe or medication to keep their heart pumping.

4.2.2 A severe form of COVID-19:

Defined by one of the following categories:

Oxygen in the air less than 90%.

- signs of pneumonia -> symptoms of pneumonia
- Signs of severe breathing difficulty: in adults, this includes using extra muscles to breathe, being unable to speak in a complete sentence, and breathing more than 30 times a minute. In children, signs include severe pulling under the ribs, groaning when breathing out, blue discolouration of the face or other worrying signs, such as inability to suck or drink, drowsiness, convulsions or reduced consciousness.

4.2.3 Benign form of COVID-19:

No signs of serious illness.

4.3. Superinfection and bacterial co-infections

Influenza and other respiratory viral infections increase the risk of patients suffering from co-infections or bacterial superinfections of the respiratory tract, which can worsen their state of health.

Some patients may die as a result of bacterial co-infection rather than the virus itself.

There is no uniform definition that accurately differentiates co-infections from bacterial superinfections, and these terms are frequently used interchangeably in the literature.

Nevertheless, it seems essential to distinguish between community-acquired and nosocomial infections, as the pathogens likely to be involved vary, which also influences empirical treatment and possible preventive measures.

Despite a lack of information, cases of covid-19-related bacterial infections are poorly documented, particularly in patients in critical care units.

The ways in which viruses contribute to these additional infections are diverse and complicated. We have a good understanding of how viruses affect the respiratory tract and how they disrupt the body's natural and acquired defences. This allows bacteria to grow, settle and penetrate parts of the respiratory tract that are normally clean.

Most patients admitted to hospital with COVID-19 do not usually require treatment or testing for bacterial infections on admission. However, it is important for doctors to monitor for bacterial infections that may occur in hospital.

Diagnosing pneumonia is still difficult because there are no simple, safe tools that can accurately identify the germs responsible. Although blood cultures are very accurate, sputum is the most commonly used non-sterile sample. However, the main problem is that it is difficult to collect good quality sputum, especially in the elderly.

Nose and throat swabs for PCR testing for Mycoplasma and Chlamydia may show carriage rather than true infection. In addition,

bronchoalveolar lavage (BAL) is often seen as the best test for diagnosing pneumonia.
However, it is invasive and difficult to perform, so it is generally only used in patients with severe pneumonia or a weakened immune system. Furthermore, during covid-19, BAL was rarely used. This is due to the risk it poses to nursing staff, the increase in their workload and the danger that the technique could worsen the patient's breathing during the procedure.
The most common micro-organisms include Staphylococcus aureus, Streptococcus pneumoniae and Haemophilus influenzae, as well as other varieties of bacteria. Although initially uncommon, bacterial infections often occur in patients who are hospitalised over a long period, particularly due to Pseudomonas aeruginosa, Klebsiella spp and S. aureus, which are common germs.
Studies have shown that high levels of C-reactive protein (CRP) and procalcitonin (PCT) are associated with severe cases of covid-19 and a poorer prognosis.
However, it remains unclear whether elevated levels of these markers in the blood of critically ill covid-19 patients indicate the presence of additional or new bacterial infections.
It appears that high CRP levels are frequently attributed to the inflammatory response induced by SARS-CoV-2. PCT may be more relevant for patients with a less severe form of the disease.
Individuals suffering from covid-19 often have increased levels of PCT, even in the absence of bacterial infection. Further research is required to assess the effectiveness of this indicator in the context of co-infections and superinfections before any meaningful conclusions can be drawn.

Covid-19 is often associated with visible lung problems on X-rays, such as areas of thickening or blurred spots. These problems are often found in both lungs and in several places.

If a chest X-ray shows signs that are not normal for covid-19, such as an infection in a single lobe of the lungs, it is preferable to think of a bacterial infection in addition and to start antibiotic treatment.

4.4. Biological signs :

The onset of symptoms is accompanied by changes in blood tests. The tests recommended in emergency departments are :

- Blood count: often shows lymphopenia, sometimes hyperleukocytosis in cases of superinfection. Sometimes there is a drop in haemoglobin and platelet levels.
- Inflammatory work-up :
  - CRP, VS, Ferritinemia
  - IL-6, IL-10, IL-2, IL-7, IL-10.
  - Tumour necrosis factor-α (TNF-α).
  - Macrophage inflammatory protein 1-α (MIP -1α)
  - TNF-α.
- Renal function
- Liver check-up
- D-Dimer, troponin
- CPK
- Blood ionogram
- LDH
- Blood cultures in case of superinfection

5. Positive diagnosis :

5.1. Biological diagnostics

5.1.1 Direct debit :

Respiratory oropharyngeal swabs are the main method used to diagnose covid-19. First of all, it is crucial to follow protocols to prevent contamination when collecting samples from an individual. Wooden swabs are not suitable for diagnostic tests using molecular biology techniques.

In general, the sampling technique is not without risks.

However, it is essential to have a good knowledge of body references:

The depth at which the nasal sample is taken must be adapted to the anatomical complexity of the nose, as well as to variations caused by congenital anomalies or sinus disorders.

The nasal cavity is a small passageway linking the front of the nose to the nasopharynx at the back. The right and left nostrils are divided by a membrane known as the septum, which is often deviated. It is quite rare for the two nostrils to be perfectly identical.

The difficulties encountered when passing through the nasal cavity are mainly due to variations in its structure, although diseases can also be the cause, although this occurs less frequently. These problems often occur as a result of hypertrophy of the inferior nasal turbinate, deviation of the septum, polyps, or nasal or sinus surgery. Major sinus surgery, such as ethmoidectomy, can make the roof of the nasal cavity more fragile, as it is no longer protected by the various parts inside. It is therefore important to be careful when taking samples and to remain level with the floor of the nasal cavity, without going upwards.

First of all, it is important to reassure the patient. Before the sample is taken, the patient must be made to understand what is going to be done. The procedure is as follows:

- The patient must be calm and seated comfortably during the sample collection.
- Ask him to blow his nose first, then tilt his head back slightly.
- You can support his head with one hand or lean it against the wall to reduce movement during collection.
- Stay close to the patient to avoid being contaminated when coughing or sneezing.
- Start by inserting the swab horizontally into one nostril,
- The swab moves gently and evenly along the floor to reach the back of the lower horn and the back wall of the nasopharynx.
- Hold it in place for 5 to 10 seconds and rotate it.
- It is important to rub gently without exerting too much pressure on the mucosa.
- The cells are picked up at the end of the cotton bud and gently removed.
- If you encounter resistance, never try to force your way into your nose, as this can cause injury and bleeding.

5.1.2 Diagnostic methods :

Real-time RT-PCR :

This test is performed on viral RNA taken from nose or throat samples, saliva or sometimes blood. It is generally carried out on patients who may be infected with SARS-CoV-2.

The main test for detecting SARS-CoV-2 infection remains RT-PCR.

Real-time PCR technique (RT-PCR) means a method for measuring the levels of DNA or RNA in a sample while the reaction is taking place.

Various methods have been suggested for finding the virus RNA using one technique.

Real-time RT-PCR is a method used to detect and measure DNA or RNA in samples, obtaining results rapidly and in real time. The real-time RT-PCR method is highly accurate and provides a reliable diagnosis within three hours. However, laboratories generally take between six and eight hours to deliver results. It is much faster than other ways of isolating the virus and has less risk of contamination or error, as all the steps can be carried out in a closed tube. The tests used to detect the nucleic acids of the SARS-CoV-2 coronavirus are based on a method called real-time RT-PCR. This approach uses a light probe and specific segments of DNA to identify two or three particular areas within the gene of the new coronavirus. These protocols differ in terms of the virus genes that are identified.

- RdRP
- ORF1ab
- Gene E
- Gene N

It is possible to detect each gene in isolation or all the genes simultaneously.

According to the WHO, a proper diagnosis must be made using tests that detect. "Two independent targets of the SARS-CoV-2 genome."

Viral RNA can still be found in the oro-rhinopharynx and in the faeces after symptoms have subsided and Covid-19 has been treated. In some patients, the RT-PCR test has been positive for up to six weeks after the onset of symptoms, long after the body has produced antibodies.

In an American study conducted. In people who were still symptomatic up to 20 days after the onset of symptoms, the SARS-CoV-2 virus could not be found in the samples.

So a positive test confirms the diagnosis, but a negative test does not.

Viral RNA can be detected more than 30 days later without the virus being contagious.

Rapid antigen detection tests (RATs)

The principle is generally based on a method called immunochromatography. The results can be read manually or automatically. Their main advantage is that the results arrive quickly, in around 10 to 15 minutes, which is much faster than the fastest PCR solutions. However, when sensitivity is below 70%, some antigen detection tests are not as effective as the PCR test.

These tests could also give false positives by identifying the antigens of other coronaviruses other than SARS-CoV-2.

A negative test does not rule out covid-19 infection, in which case an RT-PCR test should be carried out, as the level of sensitivity is fairly low.

These tests are used to identify individuals likely to transmit the virus and enable clusters of cases to be rapidly identified.

Serological tests

Serological tests are complementary methods to PCR, which can be used to detect specific IgM and IgG antibodies to the virus using rapid tests based on conventional enzyme-linked immunosorbent assays or chromatographic immunosorbent assays . Detection of these antibodies therefore indicates exposure to Sars-CoV-2.

From the seventh day, IgM antibodies begin to form, while IgG antibodies start to appear from the tenth day.

One of the problems with blood tests is that they are not very accurate at the beginning, when the body has not yet created the targeted antibodies.

Today, there are many tests available, with variable specificities and sensitivities, but high overall. The variability of results depends on the immune window. Ideally, therefore, serology should be carried out at the right time, avoiding the window period. To achieve this, blood tests for IgM and IgG should be performed on a sample taken more than 14 days after the onset of symptoms.

The presence of anti-SARS-CoV-2 IgG class serum antibodies is an indication of previous contact with this virus; conversely, the absence of such antibodies does not rule out this possibility.

The absence of an immune system response beyond 30 days in some people who have been harmlessly infected with SARS-CoV-2 warrants our attention. And these patients need to be investigated for a cellular immunity deficit.

In 2020, the HAS gave further details on the use of automatic screening tests:

- Initial diagnosis of seriously ill patients in hospital, if their symptoms or examination results suggest a problem and the RT-PCR test is negative.
- Sero-epidemiological studies as part of disease surveillance.
- Initial diagnosis of patients with symptoms but no serious signs, who are followed up in the community if their symptoms suggest a problem and their RT-PCR test is negative.
- Follow-up test for very ill patients in hospital who have not been able to have an RT-PCR test within seven days.
- Remote diagnostic tests for patients with symptoms but without severe clinical signs who have not undergone RT-PCR testing since the start of phase 2 (from week 10 of 2020).
- A follow-up test for patients who have symptoms and could be ill, but who are not showing any serious signs. These patients have not been able to undergo an RT-PCR test in the previous seven days.

- Detection of antibodies in people from non-diseased communities during screening tests, with identification of close contacts by RT-PCR, according to the rules in place after a negative RT-PCR test, only for each person on medical prescription.
- Detection of antibodies in carers who have no symptoms, during screening and detection of people who have been in contact, by RT-PCR test in accordance with current recommendations. This is done after a negative RT-PCR test, only for each person on medical prescription.

Several serological tests are available. These blood tests are a good way of finding out how many people have been infected with SARS-CoV-2 and whether or not the population has good collective protection.

5.2. Medical imaging :

During the Covid-19 pandemic, thoracic tomography is a tool for diagnosing the disease.

CT scanning has become an important tool for diagnosing and assessing pneumonia caused by SARS-COV-2. It is essential that radiologists know how to use it properly to help treat this disease.

The thoracic CT scan should not be considered as a screening test in place of other microbiological laboratory tests.

PCR remains the key test forconfirming infection with SARS-CoV-2.

However, in patients showing signs of serious illness or with co-morbidities, it is advisable to hospitalise the patient and carry out a thoracic CT scan without injections, while taking samples to check for SARS-CoV-2.

Imaging is not indicated:

- In patients who have COVID-19 but are not showing serious symptoms.

- People with other health problems that do not formally require hospitalisation should not benefit from a chest CT scan.
- Hospitalised patients with no signs of worsening breathing should not have access to new images of the lungs.

Chest CT is considered the approved imaging test for suspected SARS-CoV-2 pneumonia.

A chest CT scan is recommended in cases of severe symptoms and for patients with co-morbidities.

It is possible to obtain a negative result for the first three days following the onset of symptoms.

5.2.1 Chest X-ray:

A chest X-ray is not considered to be a good way of checking for Covid-19 pneumonia. It is useless for looking for ground-glass opacities. It is therefore not very sensitive or specific.

However, it retains its other clinical benefits, including possible pneumothorax and acute pulmonary oedema.

A normal X-ray does not rule out the diagnosis of Covid-19 pneumonia.

5.2.2 Chest CT :

The images usually described are :

- Ground-glass opacities in peripheral areas under the pleura,
- which are not organised on a systematic basis,
- asymmetrical and of a different size,
- limited to smaller or larger ranges.
- Generally, no adenopathy, pleural effusion or nodular parenchymal images are found.

Other signs observed include:

- fine lines,

- thickening around the bronchi and vessels,
- dilation of vessels near or inside the lesions,
- or signs of tissue deformation.

The way in which covid-19 manifests itself is fairly similar to that of other viral infections of the lungs. However, specific features are more often noted, such as :

- lesions on the edges of the lungs,
- fine visible lines and thickening around the bronchi and vessels in cases of pneumonia linked to covid-19.

Some patients who are infected but have no symptoms may have abnormal scan results. However, the abnormalities seen on the scan are generally less serious.

The main sign of severity on chest CT is the extent of tissue problems seen on the first scan. Many studies show a link between the radiological extent of lesions and the severity of symptoms.

The Society of Thoracic Imaging recommends grading parenchymal involvement according to a 5-stage visual classification based on the percentage of parenchymal involvement:

- Absent or minimal: (< 10%).
- Moderate: (10-25%).
- Range: (25-50%).
- Severe: (50-75%).
- Critical: (> 75%).

There are 4 stages in the evolution of lung parenchymal lesions on thoracic CT:

1. Up to the first 4 days :
   - Early stage: ground-glass opacities
2. From 5 to 8 days :
   - Intermediate stage :

- appearance of linear opacities,
- organisation of condensation,
- extension of ground-glass areas,
- confluence

3. From 8 to 13 days :

- Late stage :
    - Reduction in ground glass areas in favour of condensation
    - Reduction in linear opacities

4. Late stage (beyond 14 days) :
    - progressive regression of abnormalities.

6. Strategies for treating Covid-19 :

There are several approaches to countering viruses:

- It is possible to prevent the virus from entering the cell, provided we know the plasma membrane 'receptor' to which it binds, which is not always the case. In certain situations, this method may prove impractical, because the receptor in question is essential for other crucial cellular functions.
- It is possible to try and prevent the synthesis of viral RNA.
- Another approach is to inhibit the viral protease to prevent degradation of the viral poly-protein produced by the infected cell. This will prevent the assembly of the viral particles within the cell, thereby terminating the infection. This method has been successfully used to treat various viral infections, including AIDS and hepatitis C, although it does not completely eliminate the virus from the host organism.

6.1.1 Inhibition of SARS-CoV-2 protease :

Viral proteases play a crucial role in virus production within an infected cell, as they facilitate a maturation step by cleaving large viral proteins at specific sites.

They are specific to a particular virus and act on viral proteins, as well as on certain host cell proteins, to promote viral replication. This is why they are of great interest in curbing the spread of viral diseases. To understand how viral proteases work, it is important to know both their amino acid sequence and their three-dimensional shape. This helps to identify exactly where the enzyme acts, which is where drugs could be targeted to block it.

Coronaviruses have two types of enzyme called proteases. The crystal structure of the main protease of SARS-CoV-2, called 3CL pro, has recently been published. Its protein sequence is 96% similar to that of the 3CL pro proteases of other coronaviruses, which have been extensively studied. This protease cuts the viral protein at 11 sites near the Leu-Gln-(Ser/Ala/Gly) motifs. The second SARS-CoV-2 protease, called PL pro, is different from 3CL pro. It has a special activity that removes molecules called ubiquitins.

This could help it to influence the way in which the body's immune system reacts to infection. The crystal structure of this protease has yet to be defined.

Crystallization data has also played a crucial role in the design of effective protease inhibitors (PIs) for HIV. Currently, ten of these drugs have received approval from the US Food and Drug Administration, including the lopinavir-ritonavir combination, which has been evaluated in patients with COVID-19.

A clinical trial conducted in China involved 199 participants, 99 of whom were treated with HIV PIs, while 100 received standard care.

The results of this study show that HIV PIs offer no advantage in the treatment of patients with COVID-19. In addition, the adverse effects observed led to the premature discontinuation of treatment in 13 patients. Although this result is disappointing, it is consistent with the structural and functional differences between HIV proteases and those of SARS-CoV-2.

Another anti-protease drug used in the treatment of HIV, darunavir, is currently undergoing numerous clinical trials, although a study carried out by its manufacturer did not show any significant efficacy in vitro.

6.1.2 Inhibition of viral RNA synthesis

To understand how viral proteases work, it is important to know their amino acid sequence and also their 3D shape. This helps to identify exactly where the enzyme works, which is the target of drugs that might block it. Coronaviruses have two types of protein. The crystal form of the main enzyme of SARS-CoV-2, called 3CL pro (which is a type 3C protease), was recently published. Its protein sequence is 96% similar to that of the others.

Inhibition of the production of viral genetic material has been used successfully to treat various viruses. For SARS-CoV-2, several drugs appear to be good options. Favipiravir, a drug that works by blocking an enzyme that the virus uses, has been shown to combat SARS-CoV-2 in the laboratory.

Similarly, remdesivir, which is a pro-drug converted into a drug similar to nucleosides, prevents the SARS-CoV-1 virus from reproducing in mice and also blocks SARS-CoV-2 in laboratory tests. However, the results of clinical tests on covid-19 do not allow any clear conclusions to be drawn. Finally, ribavirin, which resembles a substance called guanine, blocks an enzyme (RNA polymerase) in several RNA viruses.

However, its effectiveness in the laboratory against SARS-CoV-2 is limited.

6.1.3 Inhibition of SARS-CoV-2 entry into the cell :

The SARS-CoV-2 virus enters lung cells by binding to a protein called ACE2 and using an enzyme called TMPRSS2. Different methods are being examined to prevent the virus from entering human cells.

- **TMPRSS2 inhibitor**

The protease TMPRSS2 is found on the plasma membrane, where it exerts its activity at a neutral pH, while cathepsin L functions in the endolysosomes, at a very acidic pH.

Serine protease inhibitors such as nafamostat and camostat are currently being evaluated for their ability to inhibit TMPRSS2 in the treatment of covid-19.

It was found that the addition of a chemical to balance the pH of the endosomes, such as chloroquine, or the use of a cathepsin blocker, prevented infection only in cells lacking TMPRSS2. In addition, the use of a TMPRSS2 blocker on cells producing this protease made them resistant to infection, even with the presence of cathepsin L. These observations show that when TMPRSS2 is blocked on the cell surface, cathepsin L in the endolysosomes cannot activate SARS-CoV-2 virus particles. This suggests that TMPRSS2 may guide these viruses towards a particular pathway, different from that used by cathepsin L.

- **Umifenovir (Arbidol):**

Works by inhibiting fusion of the virus with the cell membrane. This molecule has demonstrated in vitro efficacy against SARS-CoV-1.

Widely used in China, arbidol is currently the focus of several clinical trials.

- **Chlorpromazine :**

Is a medicine used to treat certain mental health problems. It is often used to help people suffering from severe mood swings or schizophrenia.

In 2014, de Wilde and colleagues showed in the laboratory that chlorpromazine, an antipsychotic drug discovered in 1951, could stop the reproduction of the SARS-CoV-1 and MERS-CoV viruses. This effect appears to be linked to the blocking of a type of clathrin-dependent viral input. A clinical trial is currently underway to test its use as a treatment.

- **Chloroquine and hydroxychloroquine**

Treatments initially intended for other conditions were evaluated as part of covid-19, including chloroquine, prescribed for malaria, and hydroxychloroquine, used to treat rheumatic diseases such as rheumatoid arthritis and systemic lupus erythematosus.

Recent clinical trials carried out in various laboratories, as well as research on cell cultures, indicate that a drug developed seventy years ago to treat malaria, chloroquine, could have promising therapeutic efficacy against covid-19.

Hydroxychloroquine (HCQ), has several ways of acting, such as changing the acidity inside lysosomes, blocking endocytosis, releasing exosomes and helping phagolysosomes to fuse in host cells. One or more of these means could help to combat this viral infection and reduce the number of deaths associated with it.

However, several recent studies have cast doubt on the usefulness of HCQ, mainly because of its harmful effects on the heart, especially when taken with azithromycin. What's more, the effectiveness of CQ and HCQ in treating or preventing covid-19 is now very much in doubt.

6.1.4 Other antiviral strategies

- **Type I interferons (INF-I)**

Type I interferons (IFNs) are small proteins synthesised naturally by the body in response to a viral infection. They are part of the cytokine family.

IFN-1 production can cause problems, either if it is too low or too high. In fact, too high levels of IFN-1 due to SARS-CoV-2 are linked to more inflammation, which can have negative effects on health. So it may be worth considering treatments such as type 1 interferons to control inflammation that cannot be controlled.

Initial experiments carried out as part of the TIMING project indicate that early administration of type I interferon reduces the viral load and attenuates the symptoms of covid-19. On the other hand, late administration does not appear to influence viral load or the clinical course of the disease.

- Colchicine

Colchicine is a treatment that has been used for many years for microcrystalline arthritis, such as gout, as well as for periodic illness, Behçet's disease and acute pericarditis of idiopathic origin.

Colchicine could be of interest because of its inhibitory effects on neutrophil recruitment and adhesion, as well as on the NFkB pathway.

- **Corticosteroids :**

Corticosteroids are essential medicines for patients suffering from severe or critical forms of covid-19. They should be used in conjunction with other standard treatments, such as oxygen therapy and various drugs currently used for covid-19.

It is important to note that they should not be prescribed to patients with non-severe covid-19. In certain exceptional situations, their administration could even be detrimental to the health of these individuals.

- **Hyperimmune immunoglobulins :**

Hyperimmune immunoglobulins (HIIGs) contain polyclonal antibodies, which can be prepared from large volumes of plasma from convalescents or obtained by immunisation from animal sources. They are being investigated as a potential treatment for coronavirus 2019 (covid-19).

- **Azithromycin :**

Antibiotics are common, inexpensive drugs used to treat infections caused by bacteria. However, new laboratory studies have shown that some of them can slow down the reproduction of certain viruses, including the SARS-CoV-2 virus, which causes covid-19. In laboratory experiments, the antibiotic azithromycin was shown to reduce virus activity and inflammation.

This led to research into whether it could be a treatment for covid-19. It is important to have good evidence before giving antibiotics for covid-19. Using these drugs too often or incorrectly can create 'antibiotic resistance', which changes the germs that cause infections and renders antibiotics useless.

- **The role of antibiotic therapy**

According to the recommendations of the French High Council for Public Health:

- When there are good epidemiological and clinical arguments that pneumonia is caused by SARS-CoV-2, it is not necessary to start antibiotic treatment before having the results of the test for this virus. On the other hand, if these arguments are not present, it is advisable to start treatment with antibiotics while awaiting the results of the test, as suggested by the established recommendations of the SPILF and AFSSAPS.
- For a patient with a confirmed SARS-CoV-2 infection, there is no need to give or continue antibiotics unless there is a clearly identified bacterial infection.

  The patient will be monitored in accordance with the Haut Conseil de la santé publique's advice on monitoring patients with Covid-19. If antibiotics have been given while awaiting results for SARS-CoV-2, they should be discontinued unless a bacterial infection has been confirmed.

6.1.5 Algerian recommendations:

According to instruction n°20/DGSSRH of 3 August 2021 relating to the update of the therapeutic conduct of covid-19 cases (Algerian Ministry of Health):

A. Concerning the specific therapeutic combination

- Hydroxychloroquine 200mg :

One tablet three times a day for ten days, in the absence of contraindications, is used exclusively in hospitals.

- Azithromycin CP 250mg :

500mg on the first day, followed by 250mg a day for the next four days.

This combination is indicated during the first seven days of the disease.

B. Antibiotic treatment

Antibiotic therapy is not systematic, and is only indicated in the presence of evidence of bacterial superinfection, essentially of a respiratory nature (persistence of fever beyond the 5th day, reappearance of fever after apyrexia, cough with mucopurulent expectoration, worsening CRP). This bacterial superinfection must be documented or strongly suspected (clinical, biological, radiological).

B.1. Recommended antibiotic therapy

- Amoxicillin + clavulanic acid 1g/125mg: 3g a day for 7 to 10 days.
- Ciprofloxacin CP 500 mg: one tablet morning and one tablet evening for 10 days In case of allergy to beta-lactam: macrolides or fluoroquinolones.

Injectable antibiotic therapy for severe forms and hospital settings :

- Cefotaxime 500 mg injectable: 1g/8h for 7 to 10 days.

Or

- Ciprofloxacin 200 mg injection: one injection of 200 mg by intravenous infusion over 60 minutes every 12 hours.

7. Prevention :

Since the start of the pandemic, the application of health measures has been of paramount importance in the context of prevention. To reduce the number of new cases, the combination of individual and collective measures has proved to be the most effective and rapid method.

7.1 Individual measures :

People are advised to keep space between individuals. They should avoid congregating and stay two metres (six feet) away from others in public places.

People should avoid approaching people who are ill, especially if they are wearing a mask.

It is advisable to wear a tight-fitting mask when physical distance cannot be maintained and in poorly ventilated areas.

It is also advisable to wash your hands regularly with hydro-alcoholic gel or soap and water. Using a hand sanitiser with at least 60% alcohol is a good option.

One study showed that mucus samples containing SARS-CoV-2, applied to human skin taken during an autopsy, could remain active on the skin for around nine hours. However, the virus was completely destroyed in 15 seconds when exposed to 80% alcohol.

If you cough or sneeze, cover your mouth and nose with your elbow or a handkerchief. Please dispose of used tissues immediately and wash your hands regularly.

7.2 Collective measures:

Individuals are recommended to adopt a social or physical distance both indoors and outdoors, although the ideal distance remains undetermined; in the United States, the CDC recommends a minimum distance of two metres, while the WHO suggests a distance of at least one metre.

People must comply with the containment guidelines and quarantine if they are suspected or confirmed carriers of covid-19 infection.

7.3 Vaccination :

Covid-19 vaccines protect against the disease caused by the SARS-CoV-2 virus. Vaccination is the best way to avoid serious illness and death caused by this infection. Between January 2021 and April 2022, when the Omicron variant was most prevalent, unvaccinated people were hospitalised 10.5 times more often. For those who had received the vaccine but no booster dose, the rate of hospitalisation was 2.5 times higher than for those who had had a booster dose.
Many countries have launched vaccination campaigns focusing on the most vulnerable groups, such as the elderly or those at high risk of exposure. By the beginning of August 2021, around 9 billion doses of Covid-19 vaccine had been distributed worldwide.

8. Background to the study :

This work was carried out at the Batna public university hospital (EPH Batna), which has a capacity of 120 beds. Since the start of the covid-19 pandemic, this health facility has been reserved exclusively for patients infected with SARS - CoV 2 .
The EPH Batna is divided into two Covid-19 units: a men's hospital unit on the first floor and a women's hospital unit on the second floor. It employs 187 professionals, including 52 doctors, 123 paramedics and 12 surface technicians.

9. Patients and methods:

This is a cross-sectional analytical study involving all healthcare staff working in the covid-19 units of the Batna hospital since the first case was reported in Batna, i.e. over a period from April 2020 to September 2021.

We carried out an in-depth epidemiological study of the prevalence of covid-19 infection in EPH Batna, in a special population at high risk of contamination by SARS - CoV 2. One of the benefits of this study is that it provides a true picture of the various risk factors for covid-19 infection, and also assesses the impact of this pandemic on healthcare workers.

In this study, the healthcare professionals shared the same workplace, so they were exposed to the same risk factors and the same working conditions, in particular the availability of protective means and equipment during work, and they had the same workload. In addition, right from the start of the pandemic, these staff benefited from training and awareness campaigns on the various risks of contamination and preventive measures.

The diagnosis of covid-19 infection was made on the basis of a positive PCR or a positive antigen test and/or chest imaging data favourable to covid-19 pneumonia. We excluded staff who were not in direct contact with a suspect or positive patient. A standardised anonymous questionnaire was completed for all staff .

Occupational contamination is incriminated only in the case of those who have not had contact with a covid-19 case outside the hospital, among those close to the carer, whether a family member, a neighbour, a friend,......etc.

Using these data, a questionnaire based on all the risk factors for SARS-COV 2 transmission usually described for covid-19 infection was drawn up in order to estimate the various risk factors and possible modes of transmission in the healthcare environment.

Demographic, occupational, epidemiological, medical history, co-morbidity factors, clinical, biological and radiological data were collected. This data also covered the circumstances of exposure and the source of acquisition of covid-19, the presence of a covid-19 positive case in the patient's close circle and, finally, whether or not protective measures were available, with an assessment of the extent to which protective measures were applied at work. Data were also collected on the rate of fully vaccinated healthcare workers at the date of inclusion in the study.

This data was also collected by telephone for some staff. The data was collected using a pre-established questionnaire. Participants in the survey were informed of the purpose of the survey and the reasons for it.

Statistical analysis

Statistical Package for Social Sciences (SPSS) version 22 was used for the statistical analysis. We studied the risk factors for contamination by SARS-COV 2, in univariate and then multivariate analysis using multivariate logistic regression. Only variables with a significance level of less than 0.20 in the univariate analysis ($P < 0.2$) were included in this logistic regression. The level of statistical significance was set at 0.05 ($P < 0.05$).

10. Results :

We enrolled 151 healthcare workers, with an average age of 33.9 years (20-57) and a sex ratio of 0.23. Eighty-five healthcare workers tested positive for covid-19, giving a prevalence rate of 56.3%. Eighty-five healthcare workers tested positive for covid-19, representing a prevalence of 56.3%. These included 18 men (21.2%) and 67 women (78.8%), with an average age of 33.8 ± 67.7 years. They included 31 doctors, 52 paramedics and 2 surface technicians. 63.5% of patients were contaminated in 2020 compared with 36.5% in 2021.

Most of the positive patients were women (78.8%). The prevalence of covid-19 infection was lower in women (54.9%) than in men (62.1%). Paramedical staff were most affected (61.2%), with a prevalence of covid-19 infection of 57.1%. In contrast, 59.6% of doctors and 25% of female surface technicians were infected. Covid-19 reinfection among our healthcare staff was noted in 13 people.

A notion of contact with a family Covid was found in 43.5% (n = 37) of patients. On the other hand, the percentage of hospital-acquired cases was estimated at 56.5%, of which 12.9% (n = 11) of cases did not respect the distancing rule with their colleagues who were subsequently found to be covid-19 positive (Figure 1). 45.9% of infected healthcare workers had been vaccinated.

A significant difference was observed in univariate analysis between a covid-19 infection and the notion of contact with a family case (OR: 11.94(3.98 - 35.83); P < 0.001) or a positive colleague (OR: 4.75 (1.01 - 22.26); P to 0.031), non-adherence to distancing (OR: 2.25 (1.15 - 4.42); P to 0.016) and non-adherence to wearing a mask (OR: 10.68 (1.35 - 84.43); P to 0.006). In contrast, non-adherence to vaccination (OR: 1.17 (0.61 - 2.24); P = 0.61), non-adherence to hand washing (OR: 6.75 (0.82-55.41); P = 0.052) and hydro-alcoholic friction (FHA) (OR: 1.25 (0.63 - 2.49); P = 0.518) were not risk factors for infection.

Multivariate analysis found that covid-19 infection was associated only with the notion of contact with a family case (OR: 18.17 (5.55 - 59.43);

P < 0.001) and with non-compliance with distancing (OR: 2.75 (1.16 - 6.47); P to 0.021) (Table 1).

13 patients had co-morbidities such as diabetes, hypertension, asthma, obesity and pregnancy in 0.7%, 1.3%, 2%, 2.6% and 2.6% of patients respectively.

The mean time to diagnosis of covid-19 infection was 3.6 days [1-9 days]. A second episode of covid-19 infection was observed in 13 (15.3%) patients, with an average time between the two episodes of 10.3 months (3-14 months).

Clinical signs were observed in 92.9% of cases (n: 79), while 6 people (7.1%) had no symptoms at all. Clinical symptoms were dominated by asthenia in 71 cases (83.5%) and fever in 53 cases (62.4%). Only two people presented a severe form (one asthmatic and the other with a BMI > 30), requiring oxygen therapy averaging 6 to 15 L. No deaths were reported.

A second episode of covid-19 infection was observed in 13 patients, with an average delay of 10.3 months between the two episodes.

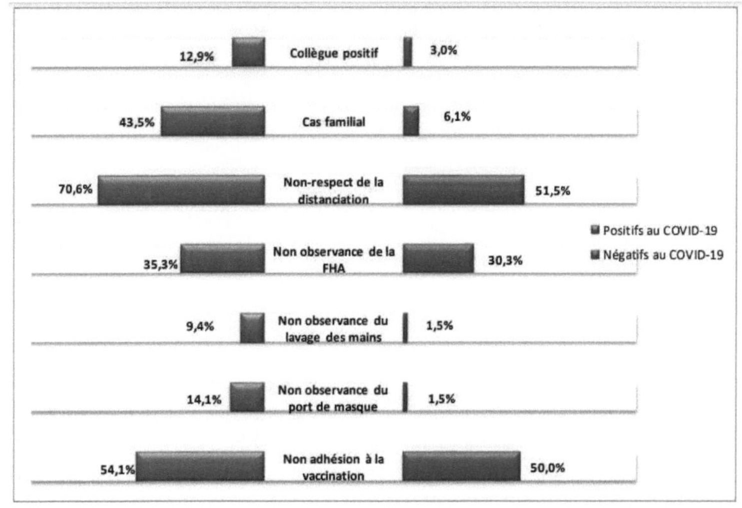

Figure 1 : Distribution of risk factors in the study population

Table 1 : Risk factors for SARS-CoV2 infection in univariate and multivariate analysis

	Analyse univariée			Analyse multivariée		
Facteurs	Odds ratio	IC95%	P	Odds ratio	IC95%	P
COVID familial	11,94	3,98 – 35,83	<0,001	18,17	5,55-59,43	<0,001
Collègue positif	4,75	1,01-22,26	0,031			
Pas de distanciation	2,25	1,15 – 4,42	0,016	2,75	1,16 – 6,47	0,021
Masque occasionnel	10,68	1,35 – 84,43	0,014			
Non observance du Lavage des mains	6,75	0,82-55,41	0,052			
Non Observance de la Friction H-A	1,25	0,63 – 2,49	0,518			
Non adhésion à la Vaccination	1,17	0,61-2,24	0,610			

Table 02: Epidemiological and clinical characteristics of patients

	Effectifs (n)	Pourcentage (%)
Vaccin Sars-Cov2	39	45,9
Deux épisodes Covid-19	13	15,3
Toux	53	62,4
Asthénie	71	83,5
Fièvre	53	62,4
Dyspnée	33	38,8
TDM thoracique	39	45,9
PCR	68	80
Test antigénique	19	22,4
Infection Covid après vaccination	8	9,4

No deaths were reported. The majority of patients had a favourable outcome. On the other hand, long covid-19 was observed in 15 patients, with persistence of some clinical signs, namely exertional dyspnoea (7.1%), asthenia (4.7%) and anosmia (5.9%).

The average length of time off work was 16.9 days (10 to 40 days). A total of 1,439 days were lost to absenteeism during the pandemic.
Of the 156 healthcare professionals surveyed, 77 (49.4%) had been vaccinated. The 60 women and 17 men had an average age of 37.9 ± 12.1 years (22-68). 42.9% of vaccinated healthcare professionals were paramedics, 48.1% doctors and 9% housekeepers.

53.2% were vaccinated with the sputnik vaccine, 11.7% with the sinopharm vaccine and 35.1% with the sinovac vaccine. 79 (50.6%) people refused to be vaccinated against SARS-COV 2. The main reasons for refusing vaccination were fear of side-effects, particularly long-term effects (n=51), young age (n=15), already acquired anti-covid immunity (n=8) and contraindications, including breast-feeding (n=5).

In our series, only 11% of professionals experienced adverse effects. The most common side effects were flu-like symptoms, fever and asthenia.

Of the nursing staff vaccinated, 8 were infected after vaccination, with an average delay of 5 months. They presented a minimal to moderate form of the disease. No severe cases or deaths were reported.

11. Discussion:

Since the start of the covid-19 pandemic, healthcare professionals have been on the front line, and they represent the category most exposed to the risk of contamination by SARS - CoV2. Many of them have been contaminated by this new virus, and others have been lost. By the end of March 2020, eighty-eight carers had died from the covid-19 infection worldwide .

SARS-CoV-19 in healthcare workers is a real challenge and a real health problem. Healthcare workers infected with SARS-CoV-2 can infect not only their family and friends, but also their colleagues and patients on the ward. This could be at the root of the considerable shortage of healthcare workers needed to care for patients infected by this virus. This absenteeism will therefore have an impact on the smooth running of the covid-19 health system.

Several epidemiological studies have assessed the prevalence of covid-19 infection among healthcare workers. In April 2020, the WHO European Region reported that of the 339,657 patients infected with SARS-CoV-2, 16.11% were healthcare workers [3]. A study carried out in China showed an incidence of covid-19 among carers of 3.8%. Guan et al showed that of the 1,099 patients who tested positive for SARS-CoV-2, 38 were healthcare professionals.

In another Tunisian study carried out in December 2020, 14.4% of the 430 healthcare professionals were infected with SARS-CoV-2 .

However, in our series, the prevalence of covid-19 infection among healthcare workers was very high, reaching a very worrying level. 56.3% of healthcare workers have tested positive for covid-19 since the start of the pandemic in our establishment.

This high prevalence in our study population could be linked to a possible failure to comply with protective measures, on the one hand,

and to the fact that there are covid-19 cases in the close circle of carers, on the other.

In our study, we found that healthcare workers who had contact with a family case of covid-19 were 18 times more likely to be infected with SARS-CoV2 than others. However, this risk increased by a factor of 2.75 if they failed to keep their distance from colleagues who subsequently proved to be covid-19 positive.

Healthcare workers are the category most likely to be contaminated. It is crucial to keep healthcare workers with co-morbidities away from the virus in order to reduce the morbidity and mortality associated with it.

In the absence of a cure for SARS-CoV2 infection, rigorous compliance with barrier measures and vaccination remain the only means of combating this pandemic.

To date, around half of all healthcare workers have still not been vaccinated, which is why we need to make an ongoing effort to raise their awareness, as this is the category most likely to be contaminated.

In our series, only 11% of professionals experienced adverse reactions. In contrast, in a study of 1878 adults in the United Arab Emirates, 64.8% reported adverse events following vaccination with covid-19. The main adverse events reported by people vaccinated against covid-19 in the latter study were: pain at the injection site (47%), fatigue and drowsiness (28.2%), joint and muscle pain (23.1%), headache (17.7%) and fever (14.4%). In another study carried out in Saudi Arabia, the majority of adverse reactions were flu-like syndrome, with fever, chills, headache, fatigue and myalgia. In our study, the most common adverse events were fever (8.6%) and flu-like syndrome (5.4%).

In our study, the reasons for refusal were fear of side-effects, particularly long-term ones. In a study carried out in Morocco, the reason for being vaccinated against covid-19 was personal and family protection. On the other hand, the main reason for non-acceptance of vaccination was lack of information and fear of adverse effects.

Despite regular training and awareness campaigns for our healthcare staff, the risk of contamination persists. This is having repercussions on the quality of the response to this pandemic, given the worrying absenteeism figures.

12. Conclusion:

Healthcare professionals are considered to be a population at high risk of contamination by covid-19. In addition to professional exposure, contamination outside the hospital remains a possibility and should not be overlooked. Rigorous application of protective measures and vaccination remain a necessity in order to protect our healthcare workers.

13. References :

1. Helmy YA, Fawzy M, Elaswad A, Sobieh A, Kenney SP, Shehata AA. The COVID-19 Pandemic: A Comprehensive Review of Taxonomy, Genetics, Epidemiology, Diagnosis, Treatment, and Control. J Clin Med. 24 Apr 2020; 9(4):E1225.

2. Backer, J.A., D. Klinkenberg, and J. Wallinga, Incubation period of 2019 novel coronavirus (2019-nCoV) infections among travellers from Wuhan, China, 20-28 January 2020. Euro Surveill, 2020. 25(5).

3. Güemes-Villahoz N, Burgos-Blasco B, Arribi-Vilela A, Arriola-Villalobos P, Vidal-Villegas B, Mendez-Fernandez R, et al. SARS-CoV-2 RNA detection in tears and conjunctival secretions of COVID-19 patients with conjunctivitis. J Infect. Sept 2020;81(3):452- 82.

4. Van Doremalen N, Bushmaker T, Morris DH, Holbrook MG, Gamble A, Williamson B.N. Aerosol and surface stability of SARS-CoV-2 as compared with SARS-CoV-1. N Engl J Med. 2020, 382(16), pp.1564- 1567.

5. Larhlid M, Manar N, Laraqui S, Laraqui O, Deschamps F, Hossini CEHL. Acceptability of anti-covid -19 vaccination by health care workers (HCWs). Saf Health Work. Jan 2022;13:S176.

6. WHO. Situation report on the outbreak of COVID-19 in Algeria.10 January 2022. [Consultéle13/07/2022].1(1):[7pages].Disponible sur : http://www.afro.who.int/sites/default/files/2022-01/Sitrep%20650_10012022.pdf.

7. Frontiers | Vaccine Side Effects Following COVID-19 Vaccination Among the Residents of the UAE-An Observational Study [Internet]. [Cited 27 Jul 2022]. Available from: https://www.frontiersin.org/articles/10.3389/fpubh.2022.876336/full.

8. Coronavirus: opinion of the French National Academy of Medicine. Covid-19: which samples for which tests? Bull Acad Natl Me 205 (2021) 435 - 438.

9. Ek, P., et al, A combination of naso- and oropharyngeal swabs improves the diagnostic yield of respiratory viruses in adult emergency department patients. Infect Dis (Lond), 2019. 51(4): p. 241-248.

10. Ahsan W, Syed NK, Alsraeya AA, Alhazmi HA, Najmi A, Bratty MA, et al. Post-vaccination survey for monitoring the side effects associated with COVID-19 vaccines among healthcare professionals of Jazan province, Saudi Arabia. Saudi Med J. Dec 2021;42(12):1341-52.

11. Lodé B, Jalaber C, Orcel T, Morcet-Delattre T, Crespin N, Voisin S, et al. Imaging of COVID-19 pneumonia. J Imag Diagn Interv. Sept 2020;3(4):249-58.

12. Xiong Y, Sun D, Liu Y, Fan Y, Zhao L, Li X, et al. Clinical and High-Resolution CT Features of the COVID-19 Infection: Comparison of the Initial and Follow-up Changes. Invest Radiol. 2020;10.1097/RLI.0000000000000674.

13. Hantz S. Biological diagnosis of Sars-CoV-2 infection: strategies and interpretation of results. Rev Francoph Lab. 2020 Nov;2020(526):48-56. French. doi: 10.1016/S1773-035X(20)30313-0. Epub 2020 Oct 31. PMID: 33163104; PMCID: PMC7604167.

14. Zou, L., et al, SARS-CoV-2 Viral Load in Upper Respiratory Specimens of Infected Patients. N Engl J Med, 2020. 382(12): p. 1177-1179.

15. Li K, Wu J, Wu F, Guo D, Chen L, Fang Z, et al. The Clinical and Chest CT Features Associated With Severe and Critical COVID-19 Pneumonia. Invest Radiol. 2020;10.1097/RLI.0000000000000672.

16. Mossa-Basha M, Meltzer CC, Kim DC, Tuite MJ, Kolli KP, Tan BS. Radiology Department Preparedness for COVID-19: Radiology Scientific Expert Review Panel. Radiology. August 2020;296(2):E106- 12.

17. Annie Ladoux, Stéphane Azoulay, Christian Dani Targeting the major protease of SARS-CoV-2 to produce an effective drug against this coronavirus. Med Sci (Paris) 2020; 36: 555-558.

18. Yang R, Li X, Liu H, Zhen Y, Zhang X, Xiong Q, et al. Chest CT Severity Score: An Imaging Tool for Assessing Severe COVID-19. Radiol Cardiothorac Imaging. Apr 2020;2(2):e200047.

19. Lambert-Niclot S, Cuffel A, Le Pape S, Vauloup-Fellous C, Morand-Joubert L, Roque- Afonso A- M, et al. Evaluation of a Rapid Diagnostic Assay for Detection of SARS-CoV-2 Antigen in Nasopharyngeal Swabs. J Clin Microbiol [Internet]. 23 Jul 2020; 58(8).

20. S. Ben Hmida, I. Bougharriou et al. Bacterial superinfection in patients hospitalized with COVID-19. 2021 Aug; 51(5): S67. DOI : 10.1016/j.idnow.2021.06.143.

21. B. Lodé, C. Jalaber, et al. Imaging of COVID-19 pneumonia. Journal D'Imagerie Diagnostique et Interventionnelle. 2020 Sep; 3(4): 249-258. DOI : 10.1016/j.jidi.2020.04.011.

22. Catho Gaud, Sogaard Kirstine K et al. COVID-19 and bacterial infections: "Current knowledge on the use of antibiotics". Forum Med Suisse. 2020 ;20(4748) :695-700. DOI : https://doi.org/10.4414/fms.2020.08634.

23. Bakaletz LO. Viral-bacterial co-infections in the respiratory tract. Curr Opin Microbiol. Feb 2017;35:30-5.

24. Instruction n°20/DGSSRH of 3 August 2021 relating to the update of the therapeutic conduct of COVID-19 cases (Algerian Ministry of Health). Instruction sur coronavirus covid-19. Available at: https://www.sante.gov.dz/.

25. Bacterial coinfections in coronavirus disease 2019 - PubMed [Internet]. [cited 12 June 2022]. Available from: https://pubmed.ncbi.nlm.nih.gov/33934980/.

26. Ahsan W, Syed NK, Alsraeya AA, Alhazmi HA, Najmi A, Bratty MA, et al. Post-vaccination survey for monitoring the side effects associated with COVID-19 vaccines among healthcare professionals of Jazan province, Saudi Arabia. Saudi Med J. Dec 2021;42(12):1341-52.

27. Ben Hmida. S, Bougharriou. I et al. Bacterial superinfection in patients hospitalised with COVID-19. 2021 Aug; 51(5): S67. DOI : 10.1016/j.idnow.2021.06.143

28. Pécheur È.-I., Polyak S.J. The synthetic antiviral drug arbidol inhibits globally prevalent pathogenic viruses. Med Sci MS. 2016;32:1056-1059.

29. Hoffmann M, Kleine-Weber H, Schroeder S, Krüger N, Herrler T, Erichsen S, et al. SARS-CoV-2 Cell Entry Depends on ACE2 and TMPRSS2 and Is Blocked by a Clinically Proven Protease Inhibitor. Cell. 16 Apr 2020;181(2):271-280.e8.

30. Dawei Wang, Bo Hu, Chang Hu, et al. Clinical Characteristics of 138 Hospitalized Patients With 2019 Novel Coronavirus-Infected Pneumonia in Wuhan, China. JAMA. 2020;323(11):1061-1069.

31. Jian Xiao, Min Fang, Qiong Chen, Bixiu Hea. SARS, MERS and COVID-19 among healthcare workers: A narrative review. J Infect Public Health. Jun 2020;13(6):843-848.

32. WHO. Available online: http://www.euro.who.int/en/health-topics/health-emergencies/coronavirus-covid-19/weekly-surveillance-report [Accessed 29 April 2020].

33. Ei-jie Guan, Zheng-yi Ni, Yu Hu, Wen-hua Liang, Chun-quan Ou, Jian-xing He, et al. Clinical characteristics of coronavirus disease 2019 in China. N Engl J Med. 2020; 382:1708-1720.

34. Chaouki Mrazguia, Haythem Aloui, Emira Fenina, Aymen Boujnah, Sonia Azzez, Amel Hammami. Infection by COVID-19 among health personnel at Nabeul Regional Hospital: epidemiology and circumstances of transmission. PAMJ One Health. 2021;4:11.

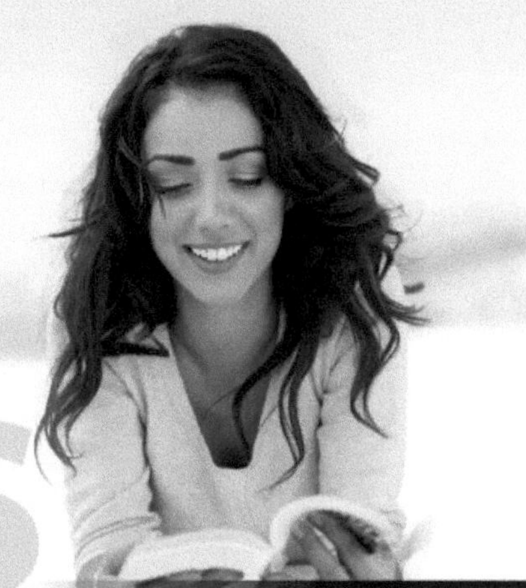

yes

I **want** morebooks!

Buy your books fast and straightforward online - at one of world's fastest growing online book stores! Environmentally sound due to Print-on-Demand technologies.

Buy your books online at
www.morebooks.shop

Kaufen Sie Ihre Bücher schnell und unkompliziert online – auf einer der am schnellsten wachsenden Buchhandelsplattformen weltweit! Dank Print-On-Demand umwelt- und ressourcenschonend produzi ert.

Bücher schneller online kaufen
www.morebooks.shop

info@omniscriptum.com
www.omniscriptum.com

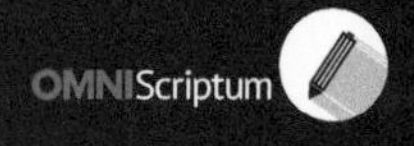

Printed by Books on Demand GmbH, Norderstedt / Germany

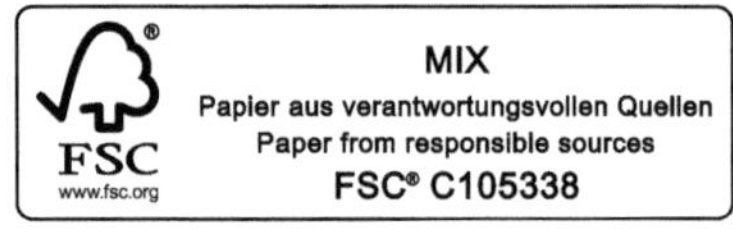

Printed by Books on Demand GmbH, Norderstedt / Germany